Rediscover You

A BARIATRIC MINDSET JOURNAL

KRISTIN LLOYD, MS, LPC/LMHC

Rediscover You
A Bariatric Mindset Journal

Copyright © 2018 by Kristin Lloyd

Printed in the United States of America
First Printing, 2018

Design and Layout by: Ascent Graphics & Design, Inc.
Published by: LC Taylor Publishings

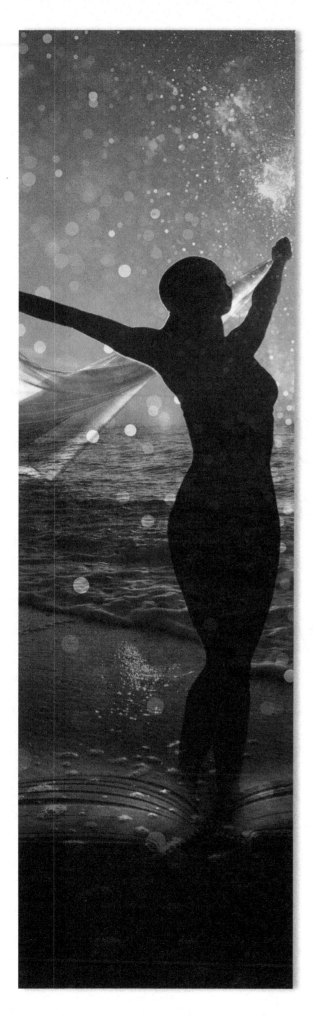

Introduction

The process of having bariatric surgery is not one to be taken lightly. It's a huge lifestyle change that occurs when you have some, or all of your stomach removed or rearranged in order to achieve extreme weight loss. In losing 50, 100, 150, 200 pounds or more, there is bound to be other things that change within you, other than the weight. Clearly, after weight loss surgery, life is no longer about dieting. It is about serious lifestyle change, and with this, comes an internal rediscovery of self, because typically life after bariatric surgery is completely different.

About 18 months after my own VSG sleeve surgery, I had to figure out who I was all over again. My body had changed, and while I had expected to be the same person, the truth was I did not know who I was anymore, or what I wanted for my life. Sure, I was the same ME, but the weight had been the focus for so much of my life, and I was feeling lost. Now that the weight was gone and I wasn't focused 900% on trying to lose weight, I actually had time to do things that I enjoyed... but wait, what did I enjoy? So, I started asking questions like, 'who am I?' and 'what do I want for my life?' along with many others.

It was then that I went through, what I call, a process of rediscovery. I committed myself not only to the lifestyle change following weight loss surgery, but also to a process of rediscovering myself all over again. I began with what I liked, what I disliked, who I wanted to hang out with, how I wanted to influence the world, who influenced me, what I wanted to do for work, and so on.

I've created this journal to help YOU delve deep inside yourself by using prompts that are out of the ordinary, and some that are somewhat ordinary to help you become reacquainted with your inner self. You might see in some ways you are the same person, and yet totally different at the same time. You might have the same values, but your inner world and the things you can do have changed, and as a result you have changed. I encourage you to use this journal to help   explore your new self, so you can live a happy, healthy, and fulfilling life in your new body with your new mindset. All while living as the NEW improved YOU!

It's time to grab your pen, a hot cup of tea (or tall glass of water), a spot in a cozy chair, and get to journaling to REDISCOVER YOU!

Are you ready?

Let's Go!

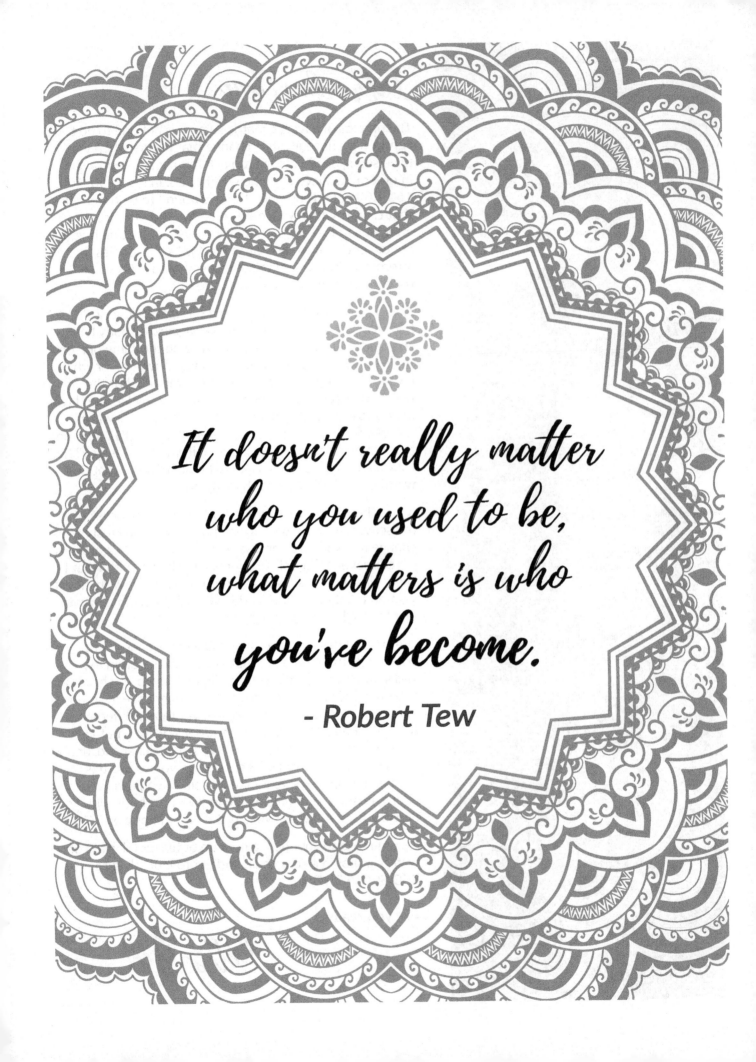

It doesn't really matter who you used to be, what matters is who you've become.

- Robert Tew

What are you most grateful for in your life (other than weight loss surgery)? Make a list of things, people, or situations that you are grateful for in your life. Why are you grateful for these things? How do they impact your life?

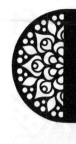

Describe and discuss your biggest life lesson to date.
What did you learn? Why was this your biggest life lesson?

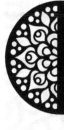

What is ONE thing you wish you knew prior to surgery
about your post-op life and why?

How has your post-op life changed you emotionally?
What do you notice about yourself, your behaviors,
and/or emotions that you did not notice before?

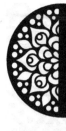

If you could do anything in your life (for work) and there were no limitations, what would it be and why?

Describe your ideal day. If you could design your IDEAL day, what would it be like? What time would you wake up? What would you do? Where would you go? Who would you be with? Design the day from start to finish and give specific details of your day from the color of your sheets, to the description of your clothes, the scents you smell, the food you eat, the places you go and the times of your events. Get very specific!

NEVER SETTLE. What does 'settling' mean for you,
and describe a time that you've settled.
How do you plan to "never settle" again in your post-op life?

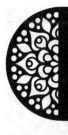

If you could go anywhere in the world, where would you go and why?

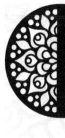

Write about a time that you were extremely proud of yourself.
What did you do? What was the situation? Describe in detail.

If you could be reminded of ONE thing daily that is positive and uplifting, what would it be and why? How can you incorporate this positive saying, mantra, or thing into your life now?

_____
_____
_____
_____
_____
_____
_____
_____
_____
_____
_____
_____
_____
_____
_____
_____
_____
_____
_____
_____
_____
_____
_____
_____
_____
_____
_____
_____

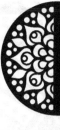

What negative thoughts do you hold about yourself?
Are they true (facts) or not true (opinions)?
What do they reveal about your underlying beliefs about yourself?

Install new empowering beliefs about yourself. List out new empowering beliefs about your life, yourself, your body, about love, about money, about being successful, about weight loss. Start with I believe: _____ and discuss your beliefs and what they mean to you.

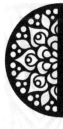

Write about one celebrity that you believe has truly
influenced the world in a good and powerful way.
What impresses you about this person? Describe in detail.

Write about a time you were extremely frustrated and felt out of control. Looking back, could anything have been changed? Would you handle it the same way? Why or why not?

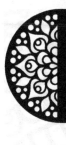

What is ONE thing you'd like to achieve in your life now that you've lost the weight that you could not have achieved as a pre-op?

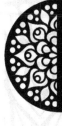

What is your favorite physical activity or workout? What do you love about it? How do you feel when you before, during, and after? What about it makes it enjoyable?

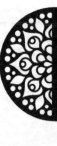

Everyone is gifted in one way or another. Describe what "gifts" you believe you have and how these "gifts" make you special and unique. How can you use these gifts to help others, help yourself, etc.?

_____
_____
_____
_____
_____
_____
_____
_____
_____
_____
_____
_____
_____
_____
_____
_____
_____
_____
_____
_____
_____
_____
_____
_____
_____
_____
_____
_____
_____
_____
_____
_____

Describe a time in your life when you've had an "unanswered prayer" and looking back, it was a blessing in disguise. What was the situation and why are you grateful that this prayer was not granted and the situation did not come to pass? How has that influenced or impacted your life?

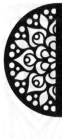

Write to someone who has never had weight loss surgery, but wants to have it. What would you tell them, and why? How would you include your own personal experience?

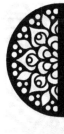

If you could take back something you said or did in your past,
what would it be and why?

_____
_____
_____
_____
_____
_____
_____
_____
_____
_____
_____
_____
_____
_____
_____
_____
_____
_____
_____
_____
_____
_____
_____
_____
_____
_____
_____
_____
_____
_____
_____

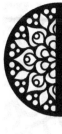

What are your best personality characteristics?
Give examples, details, and describe.

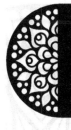

If you could learn to do anything, what would it be and why?

_____
_____
_____
_____
_____
_____
_____
_____
_____
_____
_____
_____
_____
_____
_____
_____
_____
_____
_____
_____
_____
_____
_____
_____
_____
_____
_____
_____
_____
_____
_____

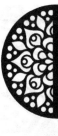

What makes you BEAUTIFUL or HANDSOME?
What do you love most about yourself physically?
Write down 5 physical traits that you love about you and discuss why.

_____
_____
_____
_____
_____
_____
_____
_____
_____
_____
_____
_____
_____
_____
_____
_____
_____
_____
_____
_____
_____
_____
_____
_____
_____
_____
_____
_____
_____
_____
_____

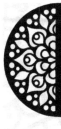

What does the term "self-love" mean to you?
How can you practice or express "self-love" more in your life?

What is one decision you made in your life that you look back on and which you wish you could have handled differently?
Describe in detail.

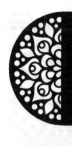

What do you appreciate most about yourself?
Describe in detail.

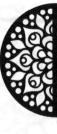

If you could meet ONE person and share several hours with them, dead or alive, who would it be and why? What would you do? Where would you go? What would you talk about?

_____

_____

_____

_____

_____

_____

_____

_____

_____

_____

_____

_____

_____

_____

_____

_____

_____

_____

_____

_____

_____

_____

_____

_____

_____

_____

_____

_____

_____

_____

_____

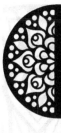

What are your biggest fears and why? Do you know where they come from? What would happen if you were face to face with your fears? What struggles have you had as a result of your fears?

_____
_____
_____
_____
_____
_____
_____
_____
_____
_____
_____
_____
_____
_____
_____
_____
_____
_____
_____
_____
_____
_____
_____
_____
_____
_____
_____
_____
_____
_____
_____

Write down your personal mission statement.
Take a look at your life, your work, your family, and write a mission statement that encompasses who you are, what you want to achieve, and what you want people to know about your life.

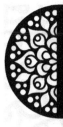

What are your biggest successes in life thus far (other than weight loss)? Describe in detail.

Go back 10 years in your past. Take a good look at yourself and your life.
If you could go back to yourself, 10 years in the past,
what advice would you give to yourself and why?
How do you think this would influence your life now?

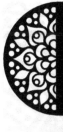

Write about your family. What do they mean to you?
What do they represent in your life?
Are they supportive, annoying, helpful, loving, etc.?

What is ONE goal you want to achieve now that you've had weight loss surgery (other than the weight)? What significance does this have in your life? What would it mean to you to achieve it?

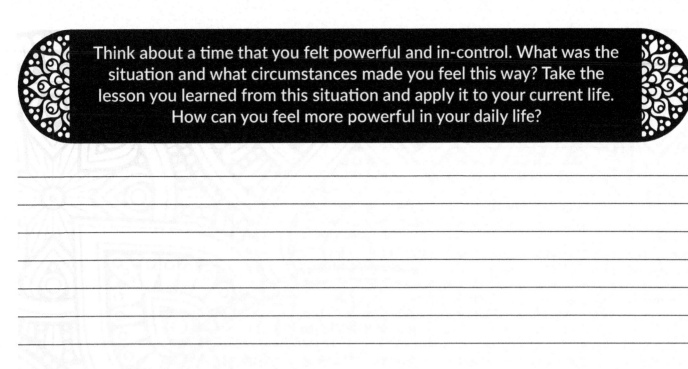

Think about a time that you felt powerful and in-control. What was the situation and what circumstances made you feel this way? Take the lesson you learned from this situation and apply it to your current life. How can you feel more powerful in your daily life?

_____
_____
_____
_____
_____
_____
_____
_____
_____
_____
_____
_____
_____
_____
_____
_____
_____
_____
_____
_____
_____
_____
_____
_____
_____
_____
_____
_____
_____

If you could only make ONE small change daily,
what change would that be and why?

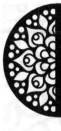

Who is your hero?
Write a letter to them and share how they've influenced your life.

If you could change ONE thing in your life right now,
what would it be and why?

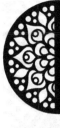

What does the word 'love' mean to you? How do you express it?
How do you receive it?

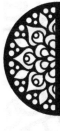

If someone were to write a book about your life, what would it be about? What's the title? What would you want them to include, and what would you want them to leave out?

_____
_____
_____
_____
_____
_____
_____
_____
_____
_____
_____
_____
_____
_____
_____
_____
_____
_____
_____
_____
_____
_____
_____
_____
_____
_____
_____
_____
_____
_____

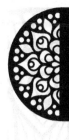

Define the word 'success' from your personal worldview.
What does 'success' mean to you?

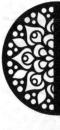

Write about something that you are super passionate about.
Describe in detail.

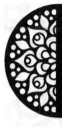

Think about a time in your life that you were disappointed.
What about this situation or person made you disappointed?
Describe in detail.

Write about a time you felt betrayed by a friend, family member, or colleague. How did this situation make you feel? If you could write a letter to this person expressing your emotions, what would you say and why?

Write down the 5 biggest accomplishments of your life. What makes you so excited, happy, giddy, or ecstatic when you think about these things? How did they come to pass? Were they goals or surprise wins? Did you have to work for them or did they come easy? How do you feel about these accomplishments?

If you had the power and could influence the world in ONE way,
what would it be and why?

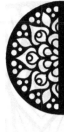

Describe your dream vacation. Where would you go?
What would you do? Who would go with you?

Finish this phrase: I LOVE _____. And describe in detail who, why, what, how, etc.

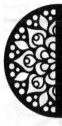

If you could be a character from a book, TV show, or movie.
Which character would you be and why?

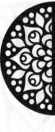

Write about a time that you were extremely angry.
What was the situation and what about it made you angry?
Looking back, was your anger justified? Why or why not?

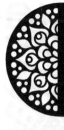

What do you see when you look in the mirror.
Describe the person you see in great detail.

Think of a fond memory from your childhood. What makes this memory special? What about this time in your life has influenced you as a person? How does this memory impact your life now?

_____
_____
_____
_____
_____
_____
_____
_____
_____
_____
_____
_____
_____
_____
_____
_____
_____
_____
_____
_____
_____
_____
_____
_____
_____
_____
_____
_____
_____
_____
_____
_____
_____

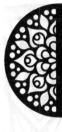

Write down 10 things that most people do not know about you.
What is it about these 10 things that make you different,
special, awesome, unique, etc.?

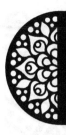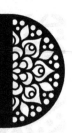

What does 'happiness' mean to you? How do you express it?
Name five things that make you happy on a daily basis.

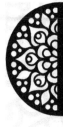

If you could have ONE superpower for 24hours,
what would it be, what would you do, and why?

Imagine that you are standing outside yourself. Write a letter to yourself about your strengths and weaknesses. Taking this opportunity to speak to yourself from and outside perspective discuss what makes you most proud about yourself and what you'd really like to see yourself change.

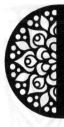

If you could TEACH on a specific topic of which you believe yourself to be an expert, what would you teach and why?

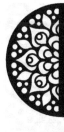

Describe the worst day of your life.
What made it the worst day and why?
How did this day impact your life?

_____
_____
_____
_____
_____
_____
_____
_____
_____
_____
_____
_____
_____
_____
_____
_____
_____
_____
_____
_____
_____
_____
_____
_____
_____
_____
_____
_____
_____

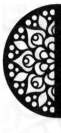

Describe a world event (past or present) that has had a huge influence on your values or world view. How did it impact you or change you?

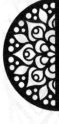

Think about your life 10 years into the future. What is your life like?
What would you like to be doing?
Who would you like to be doing it with?

Write a letter to someone you want to forgive. Forgiving is different from forgetting. What was the situation that occurred? What do you want to say to this person? What significance does this have on your life? How do you feel about forgiving them? How will it make you feel once you've forgiven them?

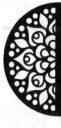

Write about a situation that embarrassed you? What happened?
How did you feel other than embarrassed?
What was it about this situation that impacted you?

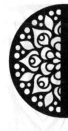

What does the word "prosperity" mean to you?
Do you consider yourself prosperous? Why or why not?

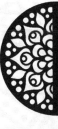

What are your biggest fears about the future?
How might you change this now so you can alleviate these fears?

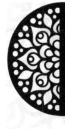

Describe a time when you were celebrated by friends, family, or by colleagues. How did this make you feel?

_____
_____
_____
_____
_____
_____
_____
_____
_____
_____
_____
_____
_____
_____
_____
_____
_____
_____
_____
_____
_____
_____
_____
_____
_____
_____
_____
_____
_____
_____
_____

Hate and Love are opposites. Write about one thing, situation or person you absolutely hate, and one thing, situation, or person you absolutely love. What do you love and hate about this thing, situation, or person?

If you could live anywhere in the world, where would you live and why?

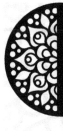

Describe the best day of your life.
What made this the best day and why?
How did this day impact your life?

Write about self-care activities you enjoy doing. What is most important to you in taking care of yourself? If you don't have a list of self-care activities, make a list of activities that would make you feel good about yourself and discuss how they can become a part of your life and integrate into your regular routine.

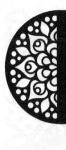

If you were deserted on an island and could only take ONE person and 5 personal items, who and what would you take and why?

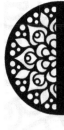

If you had unlimited money, what would you do with your life?
What would change? What would stay the same? Write a page about
what your life would look like if money were no object.

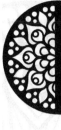

If there were a situation or experience that you could "redo"
or get a "do-over" what would it be and why?

What situations, people, or activities make you feel "worthy and deserving?" Describe a time in your life where you've felt worthy and deserving. Write about how you can utilize these situations, then create some mantras/affirmations, or create a list of activities you can do often to help you feel more worthy and deserving in your life on a regular basis.

_____
_____
_____
_____
_____
_____
_____
_____
_____
_____
_____
_____
_____
_____
_____
_____
_____
_____
_____
_____
_____
_____
_____
_____
_____
_____
_____
_____
_____
_____
_____
_____
_____

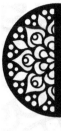

If you could change one situation in your life right now,
what would it be and why?
What small steps could you take towards changing this situation?

Write a letter to your former pre-surgery self. Tell them about who they are going to become. Tell them what they've achieved. Tell them about how you feel now, and discuss your current life in detail.

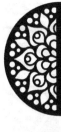

People say life is about the 'little things' because they become big things. Write down 5 little things that make a difference in your life and that add up to big things for YOU.

Notes

About Kristin Lloyd, MS, LMHC, LPC

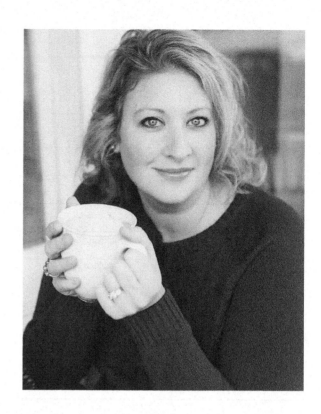

Kristin has been creating outstanding results for individuals, couples, and organizations for over 10 years as a highly-accomplished psychotherapist, transformational mindset mentor, college educator, and consultant.

Through her invigorating and transformative facilitation skills, Kristin has been guiding individuals, couples, and executives to achieve dramatic breakthroughs in mindset and motivation, self-confidence, productivity, commitment, habit-shifting, interpersonal communication, relationship renewal, conflict resolution, stress reduction, and aligning with their soul's purpose as well as reinventing one's future for success.

Kristin's passion for helping people 'get out of their own way' led her to work with weight loss surgery patients to shift their mindset after bariatric surgery. She works with them to create lasting behavioral/habit changes and emotional adjustments which lead to happy, healthy and fulfilling lives by keeping the weight off and adjusting to the multitude of lifestyle changes that occur following bariatric surgery. As a mental health professional, she is passionate about helping people overcome depression, anxiety, self-sabotage, and life stressors so they can achieve balance and sustained success through habit building.

As a doctoral candidate in Psychology, Kristin's dissertation research focus is on the process of lifestyle change following bariatric surgery. She received her Master of Science in Mental Health Counseling in 2006, and since her surgery in 2013, has combined her years of professional experience as a therapist, coach, mentor, and educator with her personal experience as a weight loss surgery patient in helping others succeed.

Having friends that have experienced regain after bariatric surgery, Kristin has made it her mission to address the emotional issues that arise after surgery to help people avoid regain, and stay on track to keep the weight off long-term.

In addition to working in a private practice setting as a licensed psychotherapist (both in office in Alpharetta, GA and online), Kristin is a PhD candidate in Psychology, a certified Reiki Master, an EFT/Energy Psychology Practitioner, certified mindset mentor and coach, a speaker, and a prolific writer. Kristin is currently a contributor for The Obesity Action Coalition, Obesity Help, The Huffington Post and The Master Shift. She is also a member of the Obesity Action Coalition.

Kristin lives in the suburbs of Atlanta, Georgia with her husband and son. Her husband has been by her side, from the beginning, cheering her on throughout her journey.

Follow Kristin and Bariatric Mindset on Social Media

 www.facebook.com/BariatricMindset   @bariatricmindset

 Bariatric Mindset   @barimindset

You can also join the email list for new information and for more information about staying on track after weight loss surgery, check us out at www.bariatricmindset.com

Made in the USA
Las Vegas, NV
23 April 2021